Green Tea for Weight Loss and Health

Detox, Boost Immunity, Lower Cholesterol, Increase Metabolism, Burn Calories and More

Kelly Larson

This book is dedicated to everyone interested in learning the numerous health and weight loss benefits found in green tea.

Copyright Act of 1976, the scanning, uploading and electronic sharing of any part of this book without the explicit written consent or permission of the publisher constitutes unlawful piracy and the theft of intellectual property.

If you would like to use material or content from this book (other than for review purposes), prior written permission must be obtained from the publisher.

You can contact the publishing company at admin@speedypublishing.com. Thank you for not infringing on the author's rights.

Speedy Publishing LLC (c) 2014
40 E. Main St., #1156
Newark, DE 19711
www.speedypublishing.co

Ordering Information:
Quantity sales; Special discounts are available on quantity purchases by corporations, associations, and others. For details, contact the "Special Sales Department" at the address above.

This is a reprint book.

Manufactured in the United States of America

TABLE OF CONTENTS

PUBLISHER'S NOTES i

CHAPTER 1: INTRODUCTION TO GREEN TEA 1

CHAPTER 2: THE HEALTH BENEFITS OF GREEN TEA 4

CHAPTER 3: GREEN TEA CAN HELP WITH WEIGHT LOSS 9

CHAPTER 4: ALL ABOUT THE "GREEN TEA" DIET 23

CHAPTER 5: SUMMING UP THE BENEFITS OF GREEN TEA 35

MEET THE AUTHOR 37

MORE BOOKS BY KELLY LARSON 38

Publisher's Notes

Disclaimer

This publication is intended to provide helpful and informative material. It is not intended to diagnose, treat, cure, or prevent any health problem or condition, nor is intended to replace the advice of a physician. No action should be taken solely on the contents of this book. Always consult your physician or qualified health-care professional on any matters regarding your health and before adopting any suggestions in this book or drawing inferences from it.

The author and publisher specifically disclaim all responsibility for any liability, loss or risk, personal or otherwise, which is incurred as a consequence, directly or indirectly, from the use or application of any contents of this book.

Any and all product names referenced within this book are the trademarks of their respective owners. None of these owners have sponsored, authorized, endorsed, or approved this book.

Always read all information provided by the manufacturers' product labels before using their products. The author and publisher are not responsible for claims made by manufacturers.

Chapter 1: Introduction to Green Tea

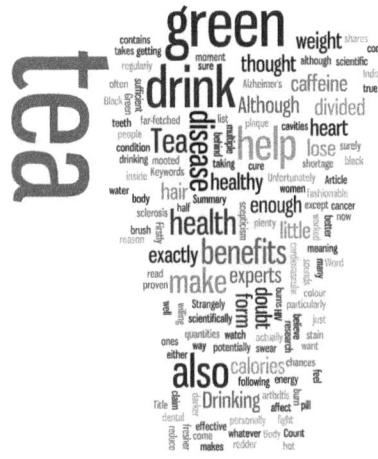

Dating back more than 4,000 years, Chinese diet green tea has been long revered as a tasty drink that can ward off diseases and improve one's well-being. Since its first recorded use during the time of Emperor Shen Nung, the link between Chinese diet green tea and good health has never been severed. It's been used as treatment for everything from headaches to depression. Today, various health benefits of green tea are constantly being reported and many scientists are now focusing their attention on the simple, yet elegantly profound beverage that is green tea.

Like all three of the major Asian teas in the market, green tea comes from the plant called Camellia sinensis. Much of the health benefits of green tea diets owe to the steaming method of making it. As opposed to black and oolong tea which undergoes full oxidization, green tea diet is only gently steamed, preserving the natural antioxidants in its original form.

The antioxidants in green tea helps fight away free radicals. These free radicals are the major contributing factors to aging as well as the ensuing degeneration of cells as a result of it. Scientists have reason to believe that free radicals also play a role in various degenerative diseases such as arthritis, rheumatism, Alzheimer's disease, and even cancer.

According to tradition, Chinese diet green tea could cure anything from headaches, body aches, and pains to constipation and depression. Over the centuries, further more health claims were made on account of Chinese diet green tea.

Chinese diet green tea is said to increase the blood flow throughout the body. Because Chinese diet green tea contains a little caffeine, ingesting this drink stimulates the heart and allows the blood to flow more freely through the blood vessels. For the same reason that Chinese diet green tea stimulates blood flow, it also stimulates mental clarity.

Chinese diet green tea detoxifies the body. The presence of polyphenols, a naturally occurring antioxidant in Chinese diet green tea, the beverage is said to combat harmful free radicals and help keep the body free from diseases. In this regard, Chinese diet green tea helps maintain the overall well-being of the body. Antioxidants in Chinese diet green tea can boost immunity, preserve young-looking skin, and brighten the eyes.

Chinese diet green tea aids in digestion and banishes fatigue. Chinese diet green tea is also said to prolong the lifespan.

For many years, men of science remained skeptical about the health claims made by Chinese diet green tea enthusiasts. Their doubt was changed to a more positive reception when subsequent researchers proved the disease-preventing attributes of Chinese diet green tea and confirmed most of the health claims.

Is Green Tea the Secret to Longevity?

That just might be.

The role of Chinese diet green tea in promoting longevity has been investigated upon by many researchers. They found the premise of their study on observing that Japanese women who are greater-than-average Chinese diet green tea drinkers; have lower mortality rates compared to others. This led the researchers to believe that Chinese diet green tea has "A protective factor against premature death."

The polyphenols found in Chinese diet green tea may be held accountable. With its high amount of polyphenols, Chinese diet green tea seems to have a stimulating effect on the immune system. Stronger immune system as a result of drinking Chinese diet green tea helps reduce risks of acquiring any illnesses.

Chapter 2: The Health Benefits of Green Tea

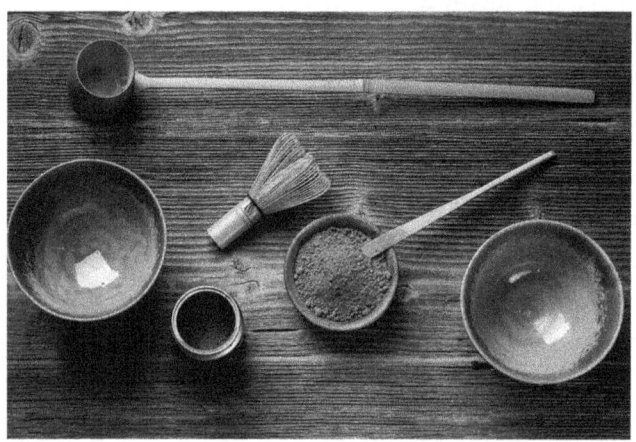

Green tea has more health benefits compared to other Chinese teas like oolong and black tea, all of which come from the plant Camellia sinensis. What makes green tea different is the process by which it is made. Green tea owes much of its health benefits to how the Camellia sinensis leaves are steamed. The steam process keeps the EGCG health benefit of green tea from oxidizing. With oolong and black teas, however, the leaves are fermented instead of being steamed, thus causing the EGCG health benefit to transform into another less medicinally potent form.

The rich presence of catechin polyphenols, particularly epigallocatechin gallate (EGCG) is the reason why green tea has so much health benefits. A powerful antioxidant, EGCG can not only inhibit the growth of cancer cells but can also destroy them without harming healthy cells. The EGCG in green tea is a health benefit substance that can lower down LDL cholesterol levels and stop blood from forming abnormal clots (thrombosis), a leading cause of heart attacks and strokes.

Aside from medicinal value, green tea can also offer other health benefits, especially in the fitness field. Drinking green tea can cause a person to burn down more calories. A recent study on the health benefits of green tea shows that the drink can help dieters. According to the American Journal of Clinical Nutrition in 1999, men who take both caffeine and green tea burn down more calories than men who only take caffeine or a placebo.

Another health benefit of green tea is its bacteria-destroying properties. The health benefit of green tea in this area is that it can help prevent food poisoning and also prevent tooth decay. The substances found in green tea kill the bacteria causing food poisoning and those that cause dental plaque to form.

Well known for its countless medicinal and health benefits, green tea is nothing short of a miracle.

Fighting Cancer

There are many health benefits associated with having a green tea diet. One of these green tea diet benefits is preventing cancer. Certain substances present in green tea diets are said to help in destroying cancer cells without harming any neighboring tissues. This substance in green tea diets is called epigallocatechin gallate or EGCG.

In the 1994 edition of the Journal of National Cancer Institute, the results of an epidemiological study stated that one of the health benefits of drinking green tea is that it can reduce the risk of esophageal cancer in Chinese men and women by up to sixty percent.

The University of Purdue has also recently concluded a research on how a certain compound present in green tea can stop cancer cells from growing.

A Healthy Drink to a Healthy Heart

Study after study has shown that drinking Chinese diet green tea and eating polyphenol-rich foods reduces the risk of any heart complications. Drinking Chinese diet green tea also helps strengthen the blood vessels that provide oxygen and valuable nutrients to the heart and brain. It has been shown that men who drink Chinese diet green tea have seventy-five percent less possibility of having a stroke than those who don't drink Chinese diet green tea.

Chinese diet green tea helps lower total cholesterol levels and improve the ratio between LDL cholesterol and HDL cholesterol. Study shows that men who drink nine or more cups of Chinese diet green tea daily have lower cholesterol levels than those who drink fewer than two cups.

Lowering Down Cholesterol

Obesity has become one of the major health issues in our society today. In fact, more than half of the American population is overweight or obese. As a result, diet and weight loss plans have become increasingly popular. But not all diet plans work. And not all of them are necessarily risk-free. A safer alternative for people wanting to lose weight are green tea diets.

Green tea diets can be a potential cure to obesity. The catechin polyphenols present in green tea diets can delay the reaction of gastric and pancreatic lipases in the body. These enzymes are actually the ones responsible for converting calories in the body into fats. By delaying these enzymes, green tea diets can therefore stop fat from being stored and prevent obesity in people.

Green tea also has the ability to lower cholesterol levels and improve the ratio between good (HDL) cholesterol and bad (LDL) cholesterol. The EGCG in green tea can stop blood from forming abnormal clots (thrombosis), a leading cause of heart attacks and strokes.

Other Health Benefits

Green tea has always been known to have several health benefits, but who knew that it could contribute to weight loss as well?

A recent study published in the American Journal of Clinical Nutrition show that green tea extract can increase metabolism and fat oxidation of the body. In theory, scientists believe that the weight loss benefits of green tea extracts are due to their caffeine content but the results of the study show otherwise as they discovered that green tea extracts have weight loss benefits beyond that of caffeine.

In their study, the researchers administered alone the same amount of caffeine as that in green tea extracts but found that it did not make any significant changes in the body's overall energy expenditure. This led them to conclude that green tea extracts have ingredients in them that actively interact with each other, promoting increased metabolism and fat oxidation that lead to weight loss.

Further findings indicated that a certain compound found in green tea extracts might be the ingredient that causes weight loss. These green tea extract compounds, called Flavonoids, may alter the way the body uses norepinephrine, a hormone that monitors how calories are burned. When flavonoids interact with other green tea extract ingredients, more calories are burned thus contributing to weight loss.

Another ingredient that actively contributes to the weight loss benefits of green tea extracts is the compound catechin polyphenols. These compounds also interact with other green tea extract ingredients in order to promote weight loss by fat burning and thermogenesis (a process of losing energy by daytime heat).

The great thing about the weight loss benefit of green tea extracts is that it does not have any adverse side effects. Unlike other herbal products like ephedra and prescription drugs for obesity, green tea extract does not increase the speed of heart rates or raise blood pressure. Not only that, but it also appears that green tea diets may act as a mild appetite-suppressant because of the presence of caffeine. Caffeine may be harmful for the body since an excess of it can cause heart palpitations, hypertension, and insomnia. However, because green tea diets contain only very low levels of caffeine, there is no danger of experiencing these side effects.

In this regard, green tea extract is an effective and safer alternative to other weight loss products which may cause harm to the user.

The study conducted by the University of Geneva on the weight loss benefit of green tea extract implicated that green tea extract can also help thyroid patients. According to dietitian Lynn Moss, M.S., R.D., green tea extract is a healthier choice for people with thyroid who may be too sensitive to stimulants. Green tea extract can promote weight loss by increasing metabolism without over stimulating the adrenal glands.

Chapter 3: Green Tea Can Help With Weight Loss

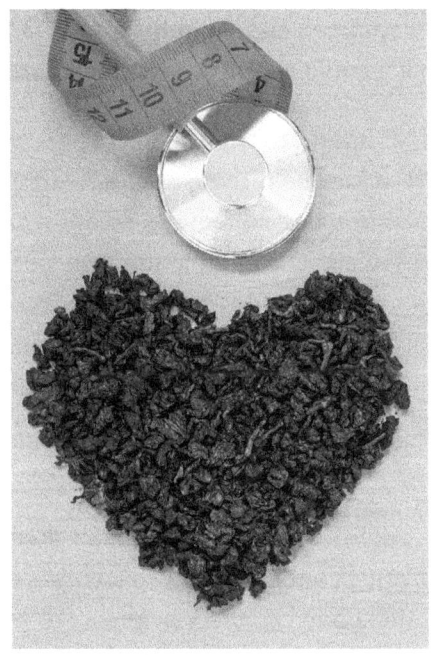

Are you in the mood for a green tea patch diet?

The hysteria on low carb diet has brought the onset of several dieting products that are based on low carb approaches. One of the newest products to hit the dieting market are weight loss patches.

Inspired by the success of nicotine patches marketers struck on the idea that weight loss patches may work the same way. Weight loss patches are basically designed for people who forget to take their regular dosage of weight loss supplements or capsules. With weight loss patches, a person will no longer need to take pills, as he will have a twenty-four hour supply of weight loss substance stuck to his skin.

Weight loss patches are commonly made from such ingredients as algae and seaweed, which are known appetite-suppressants. Later studies on weight loss and diets led to the use of green tea as a weight loss patch.

Green tea has always been known to have several health benefits, but who knew that it could contribute to weight loss as well?

Green tea is a great alternative for people who are on weight loss programs because it can help them lead a healthier lifestyle. For instance, instead of drinking coffee and cream which area high in calories, green tea weight loss programs can not only save you from taking in too much calories but also let you take in several healthful substances like polyphenols and flavonoids. Green tea also contains a small amount of caffeine, a key substance used in most weight loss programs because of its appetite-suppressant properties.

A recent study published in the American Journal of Clinical Nutrition show that green tea extract can increase metabolism and fat oxidation of the body. In theory, scientists believe that the weight loss benefits of green tea extracts are due to their caffeine content but the results of the study show otherwise as they discovered that green tea extracts have weight loss benefits beyond that of caffeine.

In their study, the researchers administered alone the same amount of caffeine as that in green tea extracts but found that it did not make any significant changes in the body's overall energy expenditure. This led them to conclude that green tea extracts have ingredients in them that actively interact with each other, promoting increased metabolism and fat oxidation that lead to weight loss.

Further findings indicated that a certain compound found in green tea extracts might be the ingredient that causes weight loss. These green tea extract compounds called Flavonoids may alter the way the body uses norepinephrine, a hormone that monitors how calories are burned. When flavonoids interact with other green tea extract ingredients, more calories are burned thus contributing to weight loss.

Another ingredient that actively contributes to the weight loss benefits of green tea extracts is the compound catechin polyphenols. These compounds also interact with other green tea extract ingredients in order to promote weight loss by fat burning and thermogenesis (a process of losing energy by daytime heat). This process is brought on by the interaction of the caffeine content and catechin polyphenols present in green tea. This is why weight loss programs based on green tea is an effective way to stimulate metabolic rates. In recent times, speculations on the use of green tea as a possible remedy for cancer have arisen due to the discovery that the polyphenol substance found in green tea can stop cancer cells from growing.

The polyphenols in green tea weight loss patches also have other uses. A study published in the American Journal of Clinical Nutrition shows that green tea polyphenols can speed up the metabolic rate of the body. With this recent discovery, several companies specializing in pharmaceutical products have started introducing green tea into the market as a supplement either in the form of diet pills or weight loss patches.

The great thing about the weight loss benefit of green tea extracts is that it does not have any adverse side effects. Unlike other herbal products like ephedra and prescription drugs for obesity, green tea extract does not increase the speed of heart rates or raise blood pressure. In this regard, green tea extract is an effective and safer alternative to other weight loss products which may cause harm to the user.

Other studies show that green tea in weight loss programs can help reduce fat by inhibiting the effects of insulin. Insulin is responsible for converting glucose into energy for the body to be stored into fat. By delaying insulin, green tea weight loss programs enable sugar to be sent directly to the muscles for instant use, thus preventing fats from forming.

The study conducted by the University of Geneva on the weight loss benefit of green tea extract implicated that green tea extract can also help thyroid patients. According to dietitian Lynn Moss, M.S., R.D., green tea extract is a healthier choice for people with thyroid who may be too sensitive to stimulants. Green tea extract can promote weight loss by increasing metabolism without over stimulating the adrenal glands.

A common beverage all throughout Asia, green tea has recently gained popularity in the West. Further researches were conducted to identify other health benefits of green tea extracts aside from weight loss. It was found that certain green tea extract compounds can significantly reduce the risk of heart disease, cancer, and even ulcers.

No supplement or weight loss program is known to work miracles. However, studies do indicate that green tea have many benefits in store for those enrolled in weight loss programs.

Sample Studies: Green Tea and Weight Loss

Green tea reduces body fat accretion caused by high-fat diet in rats through beta-adrenoceptor activation of thermogenesis in brown adipose tissue. Conducted by chief scientist J.J. Choo of the Department of Food and Nutrition, Kunsan National University, this study aimed to find out if green tea can suppress body fat and to find out whether this suppression is connected with thermogenesis spurred by the body's beta-adrenoceptor being activated.

To investigate the weight loss benefit of green tea on rats, the scientists placed their subjects on a high-fat diet and provided them with green tea extract. It was discovered that even though the rats were on a high-fat diet, the green tea extract counterbalanced fat gain without affecting the amount of energy they took in. Green tea was said to have shown some weight loss benefits in the fact that it can prevent fat from being stored, can increase protein levels, and promote thermogenesis by triggering beta-adrenoceptor to action.

Recent findings of green tea extract AR25 (Exolise) and its activity for the treatment of obesity. This study is a collaborative work between Doctors P. Chantre and D. Lairon of the Laboratoires Arkopharma in Carros, France. Published in the 2002 issue of Phytomedicine, this study aimed to find out if green tea extract has weight loss benefits and can be a potential cure for obesity.

In their study, they used an eighty ethanolic concentrate in green tea extract with standardized twenty-five percent catechins. They tested the green tea extract and were able to find that it could directly inhibit gastric and pancreatic lipases. These enzymes are the primary cause of fat storage and by delaying their actions; green tea extract therefore exhibits a weight loss benefit that can help solve obesity problems.

It was also discovered in this study that green tea can stimulate thermogenesis. Given to moderately obese patients, the green tea extract was said to have caused a decrease in weight by 4.6% and a reduction of waist circumference by 4.48% after only three months. The findings of the study clearly implicate the weight loss benefits of green tea.

Green Tea Diet Patch

The idea of diet patches is based on the marketing success of nicotine patches. Easy to apply and with no harmful side-effects, green tea diet patches have quite become latest fad in nutritional supplements.

Green tea diet patches contain a high amount of green tea extract, a beverage made from the steaming the leaves of the plant called Camellia sinensis. Green tea diet patches are said to have several health benefits. Recent studies on green tea diet patches revealed that aside from promoting weight loss, green tea diet patches can also be an effective cure for cancer and other diseases.

Clinical Studies on Green Tea Diet Patches

A study published in the American Journal of Clinical Nutrition revealed the weight loss benefits of green tea diet patches. Polyphenols are substances present in green tea diet patches that can augment metabolism. The study showed that green tea diet patches can actually increase the total energy expenditure of the body in twenty-four hours by four percent.

In addition to that, green tea diet patches seems to accelerate metabolic rates without increasing blood pressure or heart rate. Green tea diet patches promote the process of thermogenesis, a process by which the body releases heat by burning fats. This makes green tea diet patches excellent fat-burners without proving dangerous. Unlike other diet supplements, green tea diet patches do not cause heart palpitations, hypertension, or cardiovascular complications.

Green Tea Diet Patches vs. Green Tea Diet Pills

Green tea diet patches use transdermal method of delivery. This means that green tea diet patches allows the skin to directly absorb the beneficial substances, thereby, eliminating or diminishing several setbacks commonly experienced by pill users.

The transdermal property of green tea diet patches delivers consistent and even levels of substances over a period of several hours. Unlike pills which requires several applications in a day, green tea diet patches is only applied once in one day.

Ingredients of Green Tea Diet Patches

Aside from green tea extract, green tea diet patches also contain other helpful substances. Fucus vesiculosus in green tea diet patches has been used to aid in weight loss as early as the seventeenth Century. According to a recent research by Dr. Marvin Koplick of the U.S., the Fucus substance in green tea diet patches can help the body shed extra weight up to twenty pounds in two months. Fucus vesiculoscus in green tea diet patches burns fat in the safest, most effective way possible since it exhibits no side effects.

Other ingredients found in green tea diet patches are Garcinia cambogia, an exotic fruit grown in South India. Garcinia cambogia in green tea diet patches has an active ingredient called hydroxycitric acid (HCA) which is an antioxidant much like Vitamin C.

Guarana in green tea diet patches act as a natural appetite-suppressant. Guarana in green tea diet patches stimulates metabolism while at the same time, suppresses your appetite for a balanced weight loss.

Green tea diet patches also contain Chromium picolinate. This compound in green tea diet patches is essential in maintaining insulin levels in the body. With Chromium picolinate in green tea diet patches, maximum energy production, fat burning, and lean muscle maintenance is ensured.

How to Apply Green Tea Diet Patches

Green tea diet patches are applied to clean, dry skin. The recommended parts to apply green tea diet patches are the shoulders, thigh, back, and belly portions of the body. Although some green tea diet patches reputedly contain green tea worth forty-eight hours, most green tea diet patches have a twenty-four hour limit.

Green tea weight loss patches are good for people with high LDL, the bad cholesterol found in the body. Because the antioxidants in green tea weight loss patches destroy LDL cholesterols while at the same time enhancing the good cholesterol levels in the body, a balance in the body is achieved which could only lead to overall good health and well-being.

Green tea weight loss patches works in two ways. First, they suppress appetite naturally and safely. A study at the University of Chicago showed that rats when injected with green tea can lose up to twenty-one percent of their bodyweight. This is due to the fact that a substance present in green tea acts as a natural appetite-suppressant that staves off hunger.

Green tea weight loss patches also increase metabolism. With their high epigallocatechin gallate (EGCG) content, green tea weight loss patches have a distinct advantage over stimulant diet drugs which can be harmful to individuals with hypertension and heart complications.

Green Tea Weight Loss Pill

A penny for your thoughts, a pill for your fats. Who here wouldn't love a pill to melt away their fats?

People have always been known to want to do and achieve things instantly. The same thing can be said in diets and weight loss. Impatience usually leads a dieter to resort to taking supplements or weight loss pills to try to get rid of those fats faster.

Too many diet pills and products are available in the market today that it is hard to determine which one really works. Several manufacturing companies specializing in diet pills and other weight loss products are quick to claim the effectiveness of their diet pills even without proper scientific backing. Some diet pills even contain substances that have harmful effects to the body.

Diet pill ingredients like ephedra have been to known to cause complications from cardiovascular palpitations to hypertension and diarrhea. Several cases have been reported by the FDA of the harmful effects of diet pills and other weight loss products. But even then, people continue to buy and use diet pills.

Although weight loss supplements are not likely to work miracles, dieticians and weight-loss experts alike agree that most weight loss supplements greatly helps the dieter in his continuing battle for curves and muscles. Of the three commonly used weight loss supplements in the market today, green tea extract seems the most promising (the other two weight loss supplements are protein and ephedra).

Good Diet Pills

Though some diet pills contain harmful elements, not all diet pills are bad. Diet pills made from herbs can have several benefits aside from weight loss. Some of these herbal diet pills come from plants such as nettle, green tea, and dandelion.

Green tea is an herb popularly used in making diet pills. Green tea is derived from the plant Camellia sinensis, the same plant made in concocting black and oolong tea. The process of making green tea makes it different from the other Camellia sinensis teas. Because green tea is only mildly steamed and then dried, a majority of the beneficial antioxidants present in green tea remain intact.

Green tea has been known to have several health benefits. Certain substances in green tea can effectively stop cancer cells from going. Green tea's catechin polyphenols also acts as effective antioxidants that can kill harmful free radicals that cause aging. Green tea has also been known to boost the immune system.

At the University of Geneva, American and Swiss scientists were able to find that green tea has several weight loss benefits like increasing metabolism, thermogenesis, and suppressing fat intake. The results of their study became the basis for using green tea as a diet pill ingredient.

The theory of weight loss pills is based on the fact that losing weight is done in two ways: retard fat intake or expedite its burning. Weight loss pills are known to do both these things.

Diet Pills from Green Tea

Dieticians say that weight loss is achieved in two ways: reduce the intake of calories and increase energy expenditure. Green tea can perform both these functions quite well.

Green tea diet pills contain a small amount of caffeine in them. This makes green tea diet pills the perfect candidate for an appetite-suppressant. Aside from suppressing the appetite, green tea diet pills also have diuretic properties that help reduce excess water in the body. Extra water contributes to extra weight and by ridding the body of these, green tea diet pills contributes much to weight loss.

Green tea diet pills contain a high amount of antioxidants that helps burn fat faster. This claim of green tea diet pills is back by several scientific studies, including the one conducted in Geneva, Switzerland. Green tea diet pills can effectively increase metabolic rate and energy expenditure, helping the body purge out any excess calories.

The herb green tea is also compatible with other herb extracts. In fact, it is said that the weight loss benefits of green tea are enhanced when used in combination with other herbal remedies. This is what makes green tea an ideal component of diet pills.

Ingredients in weight loss pills such as Hoodia Gordonii can suppress hunger and stop food cravings. Another important ingredient in weight loss pills is glucosamine which can delay the effect of insulin, thus directly transforming sugar into energy instead of fat. Other components of a typical weight loss pill include cocoa extract (a diuretic), citrus fiber, vanadium, and glucomannan, all of which have anti-hunger properties.

Green tea weight loss supplements also contain both caffeine and the chemical epigallocatechin gallate (EGCG). When these two substances in green tea react to each other, metabolism rates increase along with the body's twenty-four hour energy expenditure. Green tea's EGCG also triggers the release of the hormone noradrenaline, an appetite-suppressant.

Green tea is a great alternative for people who are on weight loss programs because it can help them lead a healthier lifestyle. For instance, instead of drinking coffee and cream which area high in calories, green tea weight loss programs can not only save you from taking in too much calories but also let you take in several healthful substances like polyphenols and flavonoids. Green tea also contains a small amount of caffeine, a key substance used in most weight loss programs because of its appetite-suppressant properties.

Green tea weight loss supplements can boost the body's metabolic rates, thereby increasing the rate by which fat and calories are burned. Green tea weight loss supplements can also stimulate the body into burning fats faster, leading to more fats being turned into energy. According to a recent study published in Phytomedicine, a journal on the health benefits of plants, people who take in green tea extract as weight loss supplement ideally lose about two-and-a-half pounds a month.

The addition of green tea extract into weight loss pills has become common practice among pharmaceutical companies. Like cocoa extract, green tea is also an effective natural diuretic. Green tea can help rid the body of extra water that contributes to bloat and puffiness of the body.

But aside from being a diuretic, green tea is also a major contributor to fat-burning. The catechin polyphenols found in green tea effectively increases the metabolic rates of the body and also reduce food intake. Green tea also contains the substance flavanoid that fight free radicals that might be harmful for the body.

Green tea weight loss supplements come in standardized tablets or capsule forms. For best results, choose a green tea weight loss supplement that contains ninety milligrams of EGCG and fifty milligrams of caffeine. Green tea weight loss supplement is normally taken three times a day before meals. Even though green tea weight loss supplements have no adverse side effects, it is still advisable to consult medical advice before taking them.

Benefits of Using Green Tea in Weight Loss Programs

There are countless health benefits associated with drinking green tea. For centuries, the Chinese people have been drinking and using green tea as cure for several ailments. Today, cancer prevention, weight loss, antioxidant applications, anti-inflammatory and anti-microbial properties are only a few of the proven benefits contained within a single cup of green tea or a capsule of green tea extract.

Lead researcher, D. Abdul Dulloo said in a press release that there are only two ways to achieve weight loss – either reduce energy intake or increase energy expenditure. Green tea, it seems, has compounds that can increase the body's normal metabolism rate, thus giving it its weight loss benefit.

At the University of Geneva, where the study was conducted, Dr. Dulloo and his colleagues experimented on ten healthy young men. They theorized that the main contributor to green tea's weight loss benefit is its caffeine content. To test this hypothesis on green tea's weight loss benefit, they placed the study's participants on a typical "Western" diet which is about forty percent fat, thirteen percent protein, and forty-seven percent carbohydrates.

Thrice every day, the researchers measured their subjects' energy expenditure (the measurement used in determining the number of calories burned in twenty-four hours) and monitored their respiration quotient to find out how well they utilized their carbohydrates, proteins, and fats.

When they interpreted the data they collected, they found out that the men receiving regular dosages of green tea extract showed a significant increase in their twenty-four hour energy expenditure and a reduction in their respiration quotient (which means that more fat is burned, thereby achieving maximum weight loss). On the other hand, those men who were only given caffeine or placebo with every meal showed only minimal increases in their metabolism rates.

The scientists construed that the substance catechin polyphenol present in green tea adds to its weight loss benefit. These substances in green tea may alter how the body uses the hormone norepinephrine which is responsible for increasing the metabolism rate, thus leading to weight loss.

In their conclusion, the scientists inferred that green tea owes its weight loss benefit to the presence of antioxidants and the substance catechin polyphenol. These substances help increase fat and calorie burning and optimize weight loss.

Chapter 4: All About the "Green Tea" Diet

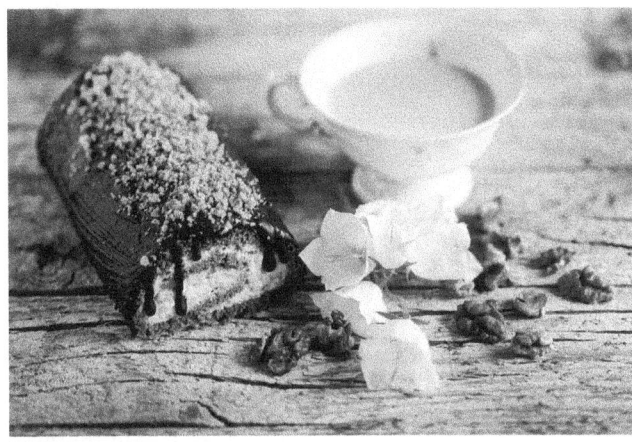

Information on Green Tea Diet

For centuries now, the benefits of green tea diets have been the subject of countless writings and scientific investigations. More than four thousand years ago, green tea diet has become a staple beverage for most Asians because of its countless health and medicinal benefits. It is said that the Chinese Emperor Shen Nung was the first one to have discovered green tea diet. Emperor Shen Nung was reported to have been boiling water when some leaves of a nearby plant fell into his pot. The leaves actually came from Camellia sinensis, the herb from which green tea diet is extracted.

Having a green tea diet is associated with several health benefits. One of the benefits of having a green tea diet is providing a potential cure for cancer. According to some studies, certain substances in green tea diet can destroy cancel cells without harming any neighboring healthy tissues. This substance in green tea diets is called epigallocatechin gallate (EGCG).

The results of the study on the cancer benefit of green tea diets were astounding and it led to further more researches that investigate other aspects of green tea diet. In a study conducted by American and Swiss scientists in the University of Geneva, it has been found that the EGCG found in green tea diets can increase the twenty-four hour energy expenditure of the body. They concluded that this is due to the ability of antioxidants present in green tea diet to stimulate thermogenesis, otherwise known as fat metabolism. According to their findings, people who were on a green tea diet exhibited a significant four percent increase in their normal metabolic rates. This led the scientists to conclude that green tea diet has a major contributing factor in weight loss.

Another study conducted in China was designed to investigate further on green tea diet's weight loss benefit. They decided that since green tea diet can significantly increase fat metabolism, then green tea diet probably would help lowering down cholesterol levels as well. Their hypothesis was proven when they introduced green tea diet on two hundred and forty people with mild to extremely high cholesterol levels. After only twelve weeks, they observed that those on a green tea diet dropped sixteen percent in their cholesterol levels.

Based on the above study, it can also be hypothesized that green tea diet can cure obesity. Green tea diet's catechin polyphenols can delay the reaction of gastric and pancreatic lipases in the body. These enzymes are the ones responsible for storing calories into fats in the body. By delaying these enzymes, green tea diets can therefore lessen fat concentration and prevent obesity in people.

A truly remarkable beverage, green tea diet is used to improve the body's health in many ways. Further studies were made on the benefits of green tea diets. The latest ones were able to prove that green tea diet can effectively protect the skin from damage due to ultraviolet light radiation. Green tea diet is also widely recognized as a substance that can protect against many different cancers such as stomach cancer, ovarian cancer, cancer of the colon, oral cancer, prostate cancer, and breast and cervical cancers.

Green Tea Diet Plan

Eating and dieting these days do not usually involve your favorite beverages like green tea and coffee. But this is not always necessarily the case. With some bit of planning and a lot of discipline, your diet plan and weight regime can include your morning cups of coffee or green tea.

South Beach Diet Plan

An idea formulated by Dr. Agatston, the South Beach Diet plan is not low-carb, nor low fat. According to its originator, the South Beach Diet plan "teaches you to rely on the right carbs and the right fats."

This diet plan is comprised of three phases – Banishing your Cravings, Reintroducing Carbs, and a Diet for Life. Using artificial sweetener and low-fat milk in your coffee or green tea during all three phases is one way to go on losing weight without having to give up your brewed cup. Going decaf with your coffee might also be a good idea since the objective of this diet is maintaining even insulin levels. If you're a green tea drinker, then there is less worries for you. Green tea contains only very few amounts of caffeine.

The Zone Diet Plan

The Zone Diet plan was developed by Barry Sears, a former biotechnology researcher at the Massachusetts Institute of Technology. This diet plan is based on the maintenance and consistency of insulin levels. Because this diet plan also concerns itself with insulin control, the issues that arise are handled similarly as that with the South Beach Diet plan. Taking decaffeinated coffee and green tea is all right as long as these beverages don't spike up your insulin. The eating program of the Zone Diet plan requires you to use artificial sweetener and low-fat milk in your coffee or green tea.

Atkins Diet Plan

Another low-carb diet plan variety, the Atkins Diet plan works best with caffeine-free coffee and green tea. For best results, artificial sweeteners in your green tea and coffee are advised to keep your carbs down.

Blood Type Diet Plan

The Blood Type Diet plan is a weight loss regimen where the foods you eat are based on your blood type. The eating program of the Blood Type Diet plan is more restricted compared to the South Beach Diet plan, the Zone Diet plan, and the Atkins Diet plan. For instance, for people with blood types A and AB, coffee is highly advised. But for those with blood types O, adding coffee to the Blood Type Diet plan should be avoided. Green teas on the other hand are acceptable for any blood types. However, adding natural sweeteners like sugar, honey, stevia, or maple syrup in green tea should be avoided in this diet plan.

Sugar Busters Diet Plan

The name of the diet plan says it all. Subscribers to this diet plan are highly cautioned against sugars. Coffee and green teas are perfectly fine but only use artificial sweeteners.

Paleolithic Diet Plan

Also called the Stone Age Diet plan, this diet plan is based on the consumption of simple, unprocessed foods that our Neanderthal ancestors would have eaten. This diet plan is perfect for green tea drinkers. Green tea is simple and one-hundred percent natural steamed dried leaves from the Camellia sinensis plant. If you're a coffee drinker, you might be in for a tougher choice since you might have to give up coffee all together with this diet plan. Sugars in green teas are still a big no-no, especially the refined kind.

AriZona Diet Green Tea

Although widely known for its various health benefits, a lot of people still balk at the idea of adding green tea into their diets. Some reason that they enjoy their coffee with breakfast and are not willing to ditch the caffeine brew for the green stuff. Still others say that it's because green tea tastes so weird.

Well, if you're one of the latter people, then have we got the right product for you! AriZona Diet Green Tea offers you all the health benefits associated with green tea without the weird taste!

Taken from the leaves of the Camellia sinensis plant, AriZona Diet Green Tea is widely known for its health and weight loss benefits. AriZona Diet Green Tea contains polyphenols which are antioxidants responsible for protecting the body against harmful free radicals. The polyphenols in AriZona Diet Green Tea helps keep diseases away.

AriZona Diet Green Tea also contains the amino acid Theanine. This substance in AriZona Diet Green Tea increases the levels of neurotransmitter chemicals that helps enhance moods and reduces the effects of stress.

Aside, from that AriZona Diet Green Tea also has great weight loss benefits. A study conducted at the University of Geneva showed that the green tea used in AriZona Diet Green Tea can increase the body's total energy output by four percent. This means that AriZona Diet Green Tea can successfully increase your metabolism, thus causing more fat to burn and helping you reduce weight.

AriZona Diet Green Tea contains less caffeine than most caffeinated drink. Medical science has proven time and time again that caffeine, though a great appetite-suppressant can cause irregularities of the heartbeat and other cardiovascular complications. Because AriZona Diet Green Tea contains less caffeine, AriZona Diet Green Tea is therefore a safer product to use.

But why choose AriZona Diet Green Tea when you can always go ahead and pop a soda? Well, for one, with the amount of calories in a soda can, it's not likely you're going to lose any weight. In fact, you're more likely to gain weight and then some.

AriZona Diet Green Tea contains Splenda, a sweetener that has zero calories. With AriZona Diet Green Tea, you get to pamper your sweet tooth and lose extra pounds at the same time. The AriZona Diet Green Tea also contains honey powder and citric acid. These ingredients in AriZona Diet Green Tea add just the right hint of tartness to the sweet drink. AriZona Diet Green Tea contains all the natural flavors that you want, plus some ginseng extract for additional health benefits.

Now, if you're the type who likes his AriZona Diet Green Tea iced, then don't look too far. AriZona Diet Green Tea also has Iced Green Tea with Ginseng Extract among its line of products. In addition, AriZona Diet Green Tea may also contain Asian Plum, Honey, or Mandarin Orange. For a more sublime taste, AriZona Diet Green Tea comes in three fruity flavors – raspberry, blueberry, and cranberry apple.

Think about it. All these fruity health benefits in a can. AriZona Diet Green Tea is green tea minus the weird taste!

AriZona Diet Green Tea with Ginseng Extract

Need an extra push to get your weight loss goals going? AriZona

Diet Green Tea with Ginseng Extract is a unique blend of green tea and ginseng extract. From the name itself, you can immediately deduce that AriZona Diet Green Tea with Ginseng Extract is a drink that will give you countless health and weight loss benefits.

AriZona Diet Green Tea with Ginseng Extract is derived from the gently steamed leaves of the Camellia sinensis plant. AriZona Diet Green Tea with Ginseng Extract has a huge following among a diverse group of weight loss enthusiasts to herbal drinkers.

AriZona Diet Green Tea with Ginseng Extract also contains catechin polyphenols that help convert fats into heat energy in a process called thermogenesis. AriZona Diet Green Tea with Ginseng Extract promotes an impressive four percent increase in the body's overall energy expenditure and can be roughly translated into a weight loss benefit of up to ten pounds a month.

The small amount of caffeine found AriZona Diet Green Tea with Ginseng Extract increases the body's metabolic rate. But because the caffeine content is not high enough to produce any harmful side-effects normally associated with caffeine-based products, AriZona Diet Green Tea with Ginseng Extract is therefore a safe product to use. Unlike ephedra, AriZona Diet Green Tea will not increase your heart rate or cause heart palpitations and other cardiovascular complications. If anything, AriZona Diet Green Tea with Ginseng Extract will even prevent that from happening.

AriZona Diet Green Tea with Ginseng Extract also contains the amino acid Theanine. This substance in AriZona Diet Green Tea with Ginseng Extract functions as a mood-enhancer and stress-reliever, thereby adding to the role of AriZona Diet Green Tea with Ginseng Extract as a promoter of good health and well-being.

Aside from green tea, AriZona Diet Green Tea with Ginseng Extract also contains another ingredient that is equally potent in promoting health. Ginseng in AriZona Diet Green Tea with Ginseng

Extract can enhance the immune system, lower down blood sugar levels, reduce the risk of certain cancers, and improve adrenal function, physical performance, and mental alertness. All these make ginseng the perfect companion for green tea in AriZona Diet Green Tea with Ginseng Extract.

Other ingredients in AriZona Diet Green Tea with Ginseng Extract are Chromium for fat and sugar metabolism, citric acid, and all-natural flavors.

Dual Action Green Tea Diet

If you want to jump-start your fat-burning ability, then Dual Action Green Tea Diet is the product for you! Dual Action Green Tea Diet is a natural blend of powerful nutrients that when used with a diet plan, has a significant dual effect on your weight loss program. Dual Action Green Tea Diet lets you work off your fats even when you're not at the gym!

Dual Action Green Tea Diet is a fast-acting dietary supplement, perfect when you're on-the-go and cannot find enough time to go to the gym. Dual Action Green Tea Diet also contains a high amount of polyphenols that when active, causes thermogenesis to occur.

Dual Action Green Tea Diet is one hundred percent pure green tea extract. Dual Action Green Tea Diet provides you with a supercharge low-carb diet. Dual Action Green Tea Diet comes in a liquid gel form for easier absorption of nutrients. With Dual Action Green Tea Diet, you can absorb the beneficial nutrients up to two hundred percent better than those found in dry tablets or capsules.

Aside from effectively suppressing your appetite, Dual Action Green Tea Diet helps increase your fat-burning ability. The high antioxidant content of Dual Action Green Tea Diet makes it an excellent thermogenic substance. Dual Action Green Tea Diet helps you reduce the presence of fats in your body by increasing your metabolism. Dual Action Green Tea Diet makes you burn fat the fastest and safest way possible!

Because Dual Action Green Tea Diet contains less caffeine compared to other diet drinks, there is less risk for you to experience bad side effects such as heart palpitations, increased heart rates, and high blood pressure. With Dual Action Green Tea Diet, you get the best out of a healthy diet.

Dual Action Green Tea Diet contains Chromium Picolinate which is essential for converting sugar into energy. This action of Dual Action Green Tea Diet helps you create lean muscles in your abs, pecs, and biceps. The Chromium Picolinate present in Dual Action Green Tea Diet also helps you build mass into your muscles. Greater muscle mass as a result of Dual Action Green Tea Diet lets you burn fat even when you're sleeping.

Another powerful ingredient of Dual Action Green Tea Diet is Xenedrol which is actually a natural blend of nutrients. These nutrients found only in Dual Action Green Tea Diet were developed by doctors in order to help you lose fat while at the same time, curb your appetite.

Dual Action Green Tea Diet also includes the potent Advantra Z, a metabolizer. Unlike ephedra, Advantra Z in Dual Action Green Tea Diet helps you metabolize fats quickly without causing any shakes or jitters.

Mega-T Green Tea Diet

They say that an apple a day keeps the doctor away. Well, we say a Mega-T Green Tea Diet caplet a day keeps the doctor away...indefinitely!

Mega-T Green Tea Diet is the newest weight loss product to hit the market. A unique blend of green tea and other ingredients, Mega-T

Green Tea Diet is the one product that can promote mega weight loss.

Mega-T Green Tea Diet includes a high amount of green tea extract that helps suppress your appetite and at the same time, increase your metabolic rates. Green tea in Mega-T Green Tea Diet contains substances that affect how the hormone noradrenaline acts.

The key to controlling the appetite is by controlling the release of this hormone first. And with Mega-T Green Tea Diet, that shouldn't be a hard task. Mega-T Green Tea Diet is a natural when it comes to suppressing the appetite.

Aside from being an appetite-suppressant, the green tea in Mega-T Green Tea Diet also helps promote thermogenesis in the body as in all Green Tea Products. Mega-T Green Tea Diet also contains chromium. Chromium in Mega-T Green Tea Diet helps prevent fat storage. This ingredient of Mega-T Green Tea Diet also increases your metabolic rates by increasing the rate at which fat is burned. Therefore, with Mega-T Green Tea Diet, you are in for some mega fat burning!

Another ingredient of Mega-T Green Tea Diet is Garcinia Cambogia. This herb found Mega-T Green Tea Diet can help you overcome food cravings and hunger pangs. Garcinia Cambogia in Mega-T Green Tea Diet, like green tea, acts as a natural appetite-suppressant. In this way, Mega-T Green Tea Diet gives you the perfect method to avoid going overboard with your eating program. Remember, the lesser calories you take, the lesser calories you store!

Super Green Tea Diet

Nature's Bounty, America's largest manufacturer of quality vitamins, minerals, food supplements, health and beauty aids, was among those who took advantage of the recently discovered weight loss benefits of green tea. They called their product Super Green Tea Diet, a fitting title for a truly super health drink.

Similarly, the antioxidants found in super green tea diet supplements inhibit the production of insulin, the hormone that stores calories into fats. With the action of super green tea diet supplements to suppress insulin, fats are readily made available, turning them into pure energy for the muscles.

Super Green Tea Diet gives you the "extra push" you need to get your weight loss goals into action. Super Green Tea Diet combines all-natural ingredients to help you achieve the body you've always wanted. Uva Ursi in Super Green Tea Diet has diuretic properties that help you maintain fluid balance in your body. Vitamin B-6, Ginger, and Guarana make Super Green Tea Diet a great source of energy, perfect for those enrolled in workout regimens. Super Green Tea Diet also contains Ginger Zingiber officinale (root) and Bladderwack Extract Fucus vesiculosus (herb).

Super Green Tea Diet is a diet pill that really works. According to some online product reviews, you could lose up to ten pounds in a month when you use Super Green Tea Diet. Taking one Super Green Tea Diet pill after two meals with a full glass of water should do the trick for you. So drink Super Green Tea Diet and start shedding fats.

Super Green Tea Diet works ideally with a workout or diet plan. This is a provision afforded to you for free because the Super Green Tea Diet includes a specially formulated diet plan enclosed in the box.

Schiff Green Tea Diet

Consider a daily workout instead of a weekly visit to the gym. Schiff Green Tea Diet provides you with the best way to work out every day without the hassle of going to the gym! Schiff Green Tea Diet, as of all Green Tea products is an all-natural diet product that helps promote thermogenesis and fat metabolism. Schiff Green Tea Diet contains no Ma Huang or Ephedra herb. Schiff Green Tea Diet is ephedrine-free so you won't experience any jittery or nervous feelings.

Schiff Green Tea Diet can also help in reducing harmful intestinal flora while increasing beneficial intestinal flora. This ability of Schiff Green Tea Diet is the main reason why it has curative effects on cancers. This is also the reason why Schiff Green Tea Diet can reduce oxidative stress in smokers and non-smokers and acts as a powerfully anti-inflammatory substance.

A single dose of Schiff Green Tea Diet has been to known to show a dramatic improvement in antioxidant levels in the body. Schiff Green Tea Diet also helps preserve good cholesterol levels and lower down the bad cholesterol. In addition to that, Schiff Green Tea Diet has anti-bacterial properties that help prevent teeth cavities.

And if the benefits listed above are not enough, further researches were made through the years. Having green tea in a diet supplement sometimes is not enough to promote weight loss. This is why Schiff Green Tea Diet comes with standardized formulation to guarantee optimum results.

Schiff Green Tea Diet contains guaranteed levels of EGCG – 270 milligrams a day. The EGCG in Schiff Green Tea Diet is used in combination with specific amounts of caffeine – 150 milligrams a day. These two substances in Schiff Green Tea Diet make this diet product something to reckon with.

Included in each Schiff Green Tea Diet package is an easy-to-follow diet and workout plan. Schiff Green Tea Diet has also made their tablets in easy-to-swallow sizes containing 225 milligrams green tea extract, 90 milligrams EGCG, and 50 milligrams caffeine.

Chapter 5: Summing Up the Benefits of Green Tea

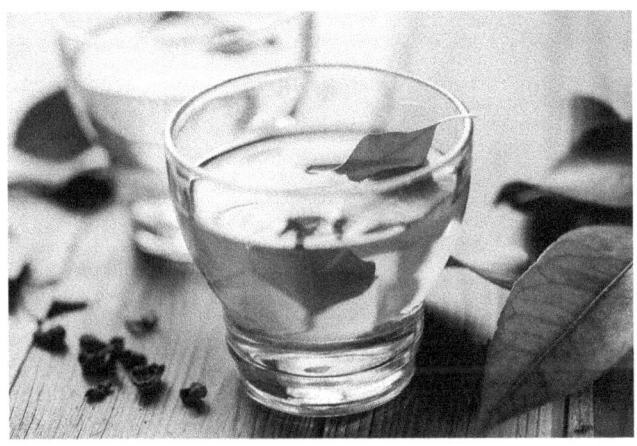

Green tea has been tested and proven for over 4,000 years starting from Ancient Civilization. Green Tea offers great benefits to the health in general. The antioxidants in green tea helps fight away free radicals which contributes to degenerative diseases such as arthritis, rheumatism, Alzheimer's disease, and even cancer. Green Tea could cure anything from headaches, body aches, and pains to constipation and depression. Green tea is said to increase the blood flow throughout the body. Because Chinese diet green tea contains a little caffeine, ingesting this drink stimulates the heart, allows the blood to flow more freely through the blood vessels and stimulates mental clarity. Chinese diet green tea aids in digestion and banishes fatigue. It lowers cholesterol level and can promote weight loss by increasing metabolism without over stimulating the adrenal glands. Chinese green tea is also said to prolong the lifespan.

There a plethora of green tea product that is around in the market now a day. These product ranges from beverages, patches, pills and supplements. It's up to you on whatever product you will use. Whatever product may it be, it can help us attain and maintain a healthy and sound body.

There is no such thing as a miracle diet. Green tea diet, like all other diets, needs a lot of work and input from those who enroll in it. Green tea diet required both discipline and heart for it to make any significant impact on your weight loss goals.

Meet the Author

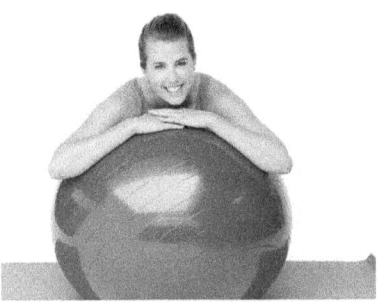

Certified personal trainer, nutrition and diet specialist and a wellness coach Kelly Larson's goal is to give as many people as possible the tools to start living a healthier lifestyle.

Kelly believes that every person can achieve the body of their dreams through fitness, healthy eating and a balanced lifestyle. Kelly follows her own personal health and fitness philosophies and believes that a "perfect body" is not a realistic goal. The importance of good health should drive and motivate people to achieve better fitness and a better body. When you take care of your body as a whole you will start to feel better and your body will transform into looking better.

Kelly lives in sunny Florida and enjoys spending time with family and friends. Kelly is passionate about music, scuba diving and new adventures. In her spare time, Kelly volunteers at her local animal shelter.

More Books by Kelly Larson

Diet Success: Nutritional Prevention and Cures for Better Health

Nutritional Prevention and Cures for Better Health: Natural Alternatives to Restore Your Health

Six Pack Abs: How to Get Ripped Abs

Stop Dieting and Lose Weight: The Ultimate Manual on Losing Weight, Getting Healthy and Changing Your Mindset about Food and Diets

Your Beach Body Transformation Begins Today: The Ultimate Guide to a Hot Summer Body

www.ingramcontent.com/pod-product-compliance
Ingram Content Group UK Ltd.
Pitfield, Milton Keynes, MK11 3LW, UK
UKHW022218230426
12048UKWH00016BA/924